99 PLUS

HEALTHY

EATING AND

LIVING TIPS

Chapter-1. 99 Healthy Eating Tips Pg. 3

Chapter-2. Other Healthy Living Tips Pg. 18

Chapter-3. Importance of Legumes, lentils and Soyabeans Pg. 26

Chapter-4. Few Interesting Recipes Pg. 31

Chapter-1. 99 HEALTHY EATING TIPS

1. Eat balanced diet.

2. Eat a wide variety of foods.

3. Eat regular meals

4. Avoid eating outside.

5. Eat meals in the company of family and friends.

6. Try to include more wholesome foods in your meals.

7. Avoid trans-fats.

8. Avoid commercially prepared foods like chips, candies, popcorn,frozen products, French fries, commercially prepared soups, sauces, dips, drinks, syrups, mixes, etc.

9. Prepare your own syrups, mixes, frozen food items, muffins, cakes, cookies, biscuits, pizza dough, bread, etc. at home level.

10. Try to use more fresh products instead of using frozen, canned or cured products.

11. Drink plenty of water and fluids between meals.

12. Try not to consume too much fluid during meals.

13. Consume your meals slowly and in a relaxed atmosphere.

14.   Do not watch T.V. while eating and pay more attention to what you are eating.

15.   Chew each bite thoroughly before swallowing.

16.   Do not force-feed yourself.

17.   Eat what you feel like eating and what is allowed for you to stay healthy.

18.   Listen to many natural food cravings and your instincts for food preferences.

19.   Avoid using salt and sugar unnecessarily.

20.   Avoid using monosodium glutamate.

21.   Avoid using preserved and processed foods containing food preservatives, artificial sweeteners, colors or flavors.

22.   Wash your fruits and vegetables thoroughly before peeling.

23.   Avoid over cooking of vegetables and fruits.

24.   Store foods at appropriate temperature, at appropriate place, in appropriate containers and for appropriate period of time.

25.   Try not to buy food items in bulk if you are not sure that you will be able to consume these within due time.

26.   Make it a habit to buy fresh and eat fresh.

27. Pay attention to all food items for their nutrient content equally e. g. fruits, vegetables, milk and milk products, meat, legumes, beans, pulses, cereals, oils and fats.

28. Add seeds and nuts into your meals regularly.

29. Avoid consuming too hot or too cold meals.

30. Adapt recipes accordingly to suit individual liking and preferences.

31. Avoid extremism in food choices.

32. It is better to under-eat than over-eat.

33. Make food choices wisely.

34.   Avoid too much intake of saturated fats and saturated sugars.

35.   Try to avoid adhering to patterns of any kind of extremist's diet plan.

36.   Avoid the influence of marketing tactics when making food choices and purchases.

37.   Eat fish regularly.

38.   Eat olives and make good use of olive oil in cooking.

39.   Make good use of fresh fruits and fresh vegetables in what-ever way you feel you will be able to consume these.

40.   Avoid too much use of fried food items.

41.   Avoid consuming too much of bar-b-q or grilled food items.

42.   Avoid intake of synthetic food supplements to overcome or prevent food deficiencies diseases, but instead make good use of all food sources in good combination to avoid and overcome these.

43.   Maintain your ideal body weight for your height and age by balancing your calorie intake with your calorie output.

44.   Avoid intake of alcoholic beverages as much as possible.

45.   Try to include food from all food groups on a daily basis.

46.   Be more practical and wise with your dietary planning.

47. Drink milk regularly.

48. Buy meat of grass fed animals.

49. Add herbs and spices in your meals for their natural remedial and healing powers.

50. Make good use of natural honey for its innumerable health benefits.

51. Avoid synthetic beverages and soft drinks and instead make good use of plain water.

52. Avoid drinking too much of coffee.

53. Avoid eating too much of chocolates, sweets and desserts.

54. Use nuts and dry fruits for snacking.

55.   Avoid skipping meals.

56.   Avoid food poisoning by storing cooked foods in refrigerator or freezer.

57.   Eat fruits instead of drinking fruit juices or smoothies.

58.   Store harmful substances away from cooking and serving areas.

59.   Avoid intake of animal sources of fats.

60.   Consume eggs regularly.

61.   Eat a wide variety of cereals and grains instead of opting just for one type.

62.   Eat trimmed portions of red meat.

63.   Avoid eating too much meat.

64.   Remember to include green, yellow and orange vegetables in your meals.

65.   Eat seasonal fruits and vegetables.

66.   Try to buy organic produce.

67.   Avoid the use of micro-wave oven as much as possible.

68.   Properly re-heat any left-overs before eating.

69.   Raw meat utensils must be washed thoroughly with soap and water before re-using.

70.   Thoroughly wash your hands with soap and water after handling meat items directly.

71.   Earthenware cook wares are the best choice for cooking as these do not contain any kind of metallic residue.

72.   Avoid using any substandard and aged herbs, spices, nuts, dry fruits and any other food item.

73.   Keep your food items covered at all times.

74.   Try to avoid any kind of direct human contact with any cooked food item if not eating.

75.   Make good use of wide variety of oils e.g. olive, canola, soybean, sunflower, sesame seed, almond, coconut, etc. to

include a wide variety of fatty acids in your diet.

76.   Make use of very mild dish washing soaps and liquids so that these do not leave any harmful residue on dishes and cook wares.

77.   Avoid using plastic containers for very hot food items.

78.   Store dry food items in air-tight containers.

79.   Do not heat oil till smoking temperature.

80.   Eat more raw fruits and vegetables.

81.   Try to consume more wholesome food items.

82.   Try to snack on natural food items.

83.   In cold weather try to consume more hot energizing fluids and food items to keep your body energized and warm.

84.   In hot weather consume more cold fluids and food items to help your body get some relief from the outside heat.

85.   Make good use of garlic, ginger and lemon in daily cookery.

86.   Simplify your recipes and cooking procedures for more wholesome products.

87.   Protect your foods from pets and pests.

88.   Try not to mix raw food with cooked food.

89.   Store cooked foods in proper containers and cover them properly.

90.   Try to grow your own produce of fresh vegetable by having a Kitchen garden.

91.   Try to avoid imported food items.

92.   Make your food more appealing to the eye by good use of different colored vegetables.

93.   While cooking your food try to enhance and create good aroma to trigger your appetite.

94.   Pay attention to develop interesting and appealing consistency of cooked food items.

95.   Be creative while cooking and use your natural food balancing and combination skills to bring out the best results.

96.   Before meals try to consume some whole fruits of your liking.

97.   Learn to develop more culinary skills and cook better food at home level.

98.   While cooking, be very careful of cleanliness and hygiene.

99.   Use good quality water for cooking.

Chapter-2. OTHER HEALTHY LIVING TIPS

•   In order to stay in a constant state of being free from illness and injury, we need to develop more discipline in life and live a life that will help us to stay in peak physical, mental and spiritual condition. More attention is needed towards what needed to be eaten and what avoided and how much activity is needed on daily basis and dealing properly with over all life approaches.

•   To achieve good health and well-being, be vigilant for all sorts of unhealthy patterns which may lead us towards chronic diseases, unnecessary weight gain, accidents or incidences of catching infections. Give more time in understanding yourself better. Have good vision for your health.

•   It is our responsibility towards our-self to keep our body, soul and mind in peak condition and free from all diseases. Clarity and strength of mind comes by keeping our physical as well as emotional health in good condition. To achieve these we need to look into all aspects and reasons behind these.

• We need to look into various reasons leading us towards emotional instability and try to overcome these by addressing them at the grass root level. Balance is needed in all areas of our life for over-all health and well-being. Imbalances could lead to disaster and needed to be tackled at early stages only.

• Imbalances at any point and any sphere dealing with health may leave negative marks which could impact over-all health. Better alternatives are needed to overcome these for more beneficial health conditions. Until and unless we learn and gain vision of what good health means and stick with the right choices we may not be able to achieve balance in all areas needed.

• Experimenting on our body by applying all the available resources un-wisely could lead towards a road of disaster which may affect our health negatively. Wise decision making is crucial when dealing with matters of health to overcome the miseries and achieving success.

• Thinking in all directions while dealing with health matters can leave lasting marks on health which could either be positive or negative depending on the choices made. An insight into the depth of the matter is needed for good results. Adopting one and neglecting others will not be able to bring much fruitful results.

• Healthy living and healthy life style choices helps in making the life more easier by allowing people to live more fulfilled and contented life. They are better able to achieve more and better through their lives while making them more capable of achieving success through independent means.

- Healthy living style helps in making the best use of ones capabilities and potentials. It enhances people's self-confidence by better results achieved through healthier living pattern. It promotes self-awareness and means of gaining good health in any given circumstances.

- One need to know and fully understand the meaning of healthy living and all the aspects and related areas it deals with. It helps in making people more productive and resilient to many difficult paths, therefore these need not be ignored if we want to achieve good results from our life.

- Due considerations needed to be given to make lifelong changes for best possible outcome in order to stay healthy and to prolong life. Eating a well-balanced diet, getting enough rest and sleep, increasing physical activity and avoiding factors leading towards more stress-full and depressive life are all important for healthy living.

• Deep understanding of the foundations and basis of good health and healthy living may be helpful in avoiding and preventing many diseases leading towards unhealthier, less productive and un-contented life. Good understanding of the factors leading towards many chronic diseases, obesity and sources of depression needed to be looked into.

• To lead a more beneficial healthy life, one need to get aware of the root causes for healthier as well as unhealthier living choices available while sticking with only the healthier ones and possible changes needed to move towards healthier living.

•   Staying mentally active has been found to be beneficial and emotionally rewarding. People who love to stay mentally active have less chances of developing Alzheimer's. There is no age for learning which is a continuous process and helps in improving mental capabilities and capacities.

•   Learning helps in keeping the mental health at peak condition and learning through reading is the most practical and easier way of giving an exercise to brain by people belonging to all age group. More challenging topic selection for learning will help in boosting mental capacity

•   Good mental health is very important for overall good health as all our body systems are dependent on our brain function and signals sent by it. Therefore our brain has total influence on the working of all our body systems. Brain health is important for over all good health.

- Giving due attention to our brain and keeping it healthy, free from all kind of diseases will need in-depth understanding of its working. Positive thinking and optimism helps in improving brain function and its capacity. All decision making should be based on this approach and the outcome needed to be handled with positivity.

- Besides optimism, a well-balanced and nutritious diet, enhanced mental challenging conditions, and proper handling of routine stress may contribute towards, good mental capacities and capabilities.

- Sharing and caring and being respectful of individual differences helps in gaining insight leading towards more happy moments and better relationships. Socialization in its true sense helps in leaving positive marks on healthy living and all good gestures needed to be reciprocated in order to gain emotional strength and stability.

- Solving puzzles and instigating various approaches leading towards better and enhanced mental exercises are also helpful for overall good mental health. Any game or activity which engages the mind to work an extra mile helps in strengthening mental power by keeping more active, productive and well occupied.

- Keeping close to people who make you happy, enrich your life, are a source of contentment, contribute positively towards good mental health. Discuss with them your worries, fears, and thoughts. Share your good times with them and become a source of happiness for them. Try to be in the company of people you like and feel comfortable with.

- True happiness is very important for overall good mental and physical health. Keeping a close contact with friends and family is helpful in keeping one happier, contented and living a life that is more meaningful. Understand yourself better and then try to understand others better so that you find harmony towards the road of healthy living.

Chapter-3. IMPORTANCE OF KIDNEY BEANS, LENTILS AND SOYBEANS

Kidney beans, lentils and soybeans come under 'beans and legumes' category of food items and are most versatile food items and provide high quality nourishment at comparatively low cost. These are low in total fat and calories while being high in over-all nourishment. These are excellent sources of high quality plant protein, complex carbohydrates, vitamins, minerals and soluble and in-soluble fiber.

The nutritional content of these foods aids in controlling several chronic diseases and reduces the risk factors associated with diabetes, coronary heart disease, osteoporosis, obesity, chronic constipation, memory loss, migraine, high blood pressure, arthritis, etc.

These are edible seeds that grow in pods and can be used to replace or substitute beef, mutton, poultry, fish and other sources of animal protein. If these are consumed in a combination and great variety with grains, cereals and several different types of beans and legumes, can help in providing low-cost essential amino acids needed for growth, repair and maintenance of body functions.

These are cholesterol free and low in fats and carry a potential to substitute meat completely and can be used in a variety of ways. Great recipes can be created and developed to incorporate these to enhance and improve the nutritional content, texture, aroma, appeal, color and flavor of cooked meals. An eye of an enthusiast and innovative ideas are needed to make it a routine meal item.

These are easy to store and prepare and are available the whole year around. In order to prevent many chronic diseases prevalent all around the world, these needed to be part of a regular diet. These are highly nutritious and cost effective food items and due to this needs extra consideration for their good humble existence and over-all goodness which has been over-looked for quite some-time.

NUTRITIONAL CONTENT

These are nutritionally dense, low in calories and rich in high quality plant protein. These are also good sources of B-Complex Vitamins, Iron, Manganese, Copper, Phosphorus, Potassium, Magnesium and soluble and in-soluble Fiber.

These are low in fat and sodium and are cholesterol free.

Soybeans are also rich in Omega-3 fatty acids, Molybdenum, Vitamin K, Flavonoids and Phenolic acid.

HEALTH BENEFITS

- Helps in lowering serum cholesterol level.

- Provide adequate amount of high quality plant protein.

- Helps in maintaining serum sugar level

- Works as a detoxifying agent.

- Helps in maintaining ideal body weight for height and age.

- Helps in regularizing bowel movement.

- Helps in reducing risk factors associated with coronary heart diseases and cardiovascular diseases.

- Maintains your memory.

- Helps in preventing iron deficiency anemia.

PREPARATION AND COOKING TECHNIQUES

- Sort and remove stones and extra material before soaking.

- Wash three times to remove any dirt.

- Soak for 2-12 hours before cooking; add a pinch of baking powder and 1 tablespoon of lemon juice or vinegar to help detoxify it.

- Strain and wash again.

- Cook in extra water till boiling point for at-least ten minutes (do not add salt or any kind of acid).

- Simmer, cover and cook till it gets tender.

- Add herbs and spices and cook according to individual liking.

MARKET PRICE

Kidney beans, lentils and soybeans all come under cost effective highly nutritious food items and the actual prices may vary from place to place and from time to time. On the average their prices may vary from 1$ per pound to 5$ per pound. Market prices may fluctuate according to production and consumption pattern of any given area. But at any given time, these are good, low cost substitutes for meat and animal sources of protein.

Chapter-4. FEW INTERESTING RECIPES

1. Beef Fried Kebabs

These kebabs are easy to prepare and store and are high in calories and protein and can be frozen for future use.

Servings: 3-4

Preparation time: 10 minutes

cooking time: 20 minutes

Ingredients:

1lb. Beef, veal, mutton, fish or chicken (boneless)

2-3 Onion

1 C Coriander leaves

3-4 Green chilies

½ C Fresh mint leaves

3 Tablespoon Ginger garlic paste (or 1 inch piece ginger and ten cloves garlic)

2 Tablespoon Lemon juice

½ Teaspoon Mustard powder

1 Tablespoon whole Cumin seeds

1 Tablespoon whole Coriander seeds

Salt to taste

Oil for frying

Instructions:

1.   Except oil, chop all the ingredients together in a chopper or food processor.

2.   Take a little chopped matter and flatten between your palms to make a round disc of around 2 inch to 3 inch in diameter and ¼ to ½ inch thick.

3.   Shallow fry these kebabs from both sides till golden brown.

4.   Serve hot with rice, sauces and salad of your choice.

2. Chicken Karahi

Karahi gosht (gosht means meat) is usually cooked and served in a karahi (round based pan with handles on both sides). This dish is very easy to cook and is rich in flavor, aroma and appeal. It should be consumed occasionally due to its high caloric value. It tastes best when eaten with a freshly baked nan or freshly cooked onion or garlic rice. A little variation in ingredients and cooking procedure to adapt individual likes and dislikes and tolerances and intolerances is recommended for overall benefit for individual use. It is a Pakistani dish which usually is eaten on special occasions.

Servings: 3-4

Preparation time: 10 minutes

cooking time: 20 minutes

Ingredients:

1 C Onion (finely sliced)

3 Tablespoon Ginger garlic paste

1 lb. Chicken (small pieces)

3 C Tomatoes (chopped)

6-8 Green chilies (cut each into two or three pieces)

1 C Fresh coriander leaves (chopped)

1 Teaspoon Turmeric powder

1 Teaspoon Garam masala powder (hot spice powder or five spice powder or all spice powder)

1C Oil

Salt according to taste

Instructions:

1. Heat oil and fry onion slices till light golden brown.

2. Add ginger and garlic paste and mix.

3. Wash chicken and drain out extra water.

4. Add chicken and fry for five minutes.

5. Add chopped tomatoes, green chilies, coriander leaves, salt and all the spices.

6. Simmer and let it cook for ten to fifteen more minutes.

7. Serve hot with rice, bread slices, chapatti, pita bread or nan and

     enjoy.

3. Khawsuey

This dish was originated from Burma and is also known as Burmese dish. It is being liked and consumed in various neighboring countries and recipes have been adapted to suit the general population of these people.

Servings: 4

Preparation time: 15 minute
Cook time: 15-30 minutes.

Ingredients:

1 packet Spaghetti (boiled, strained)

Fresh coriander leaves, lemon slices and mint leaves for garnishing

'For meat gravy'

1 lb. Beef, chicken or veal (boneless, cut in small cubes)

2C Onion (finely sliced)

4 Tablespoons Desiccated coconut or 1 C Coconut milk

4 Tablespoons Ginger and garlic paste

1Teaspoon each turmeric powder, cumin seeds powder, coriander seeds powder, red chili powder, garam masala powder, salt

3 Tablespoon lemon juice

½C Oil

'For coconut milk curry'

1 C Coconut milk

1 C Yogurt

¼ C Gram powder

½ Teaspoon Turmeric powder

1 Onion (finely sliced)

1 Egg

¼C Oil

Salt to taste

Instructions:

1. Prepare meat gravy and fry onion in oil till golden brown.

2. Add ginger garlic paste, coconut powder, all spices and meat and fry for few minutes.

3. Add little water to make the meat tender, simmer, cover and let it cook till meat gets tender.

4. In a separate pan prepare coconut curry and fry sliced onion till golden brown.

5. Blend rest of the ingredients in a blender and add little water to make it little thin.

6. Add this blended mixture into fried onion and increase the flame. Keep stirring as it starts to thicken.

7. Simmer, cover and cook for five to ten minutes.

8. Spread boiled spaghetti evenly in a serving dish. Warm it up in the micro-wave oven.

9. Add coconut curry on top of spaghetti.

10. Add meat gravy on top of coconut curry.

11.   Garnish with freshly chopped coriander leaves and mint leaves.

12.   Serve hot.